MASSAGE

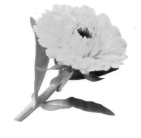

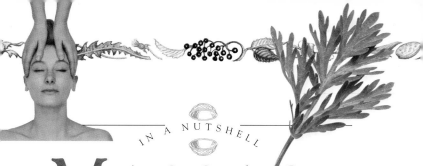

IN A NUTSHELL

MASSAGE
A STEP-BY-STEP
GUIDE

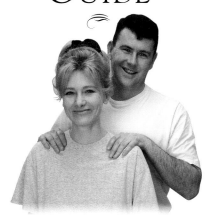

YVONNE WORTH

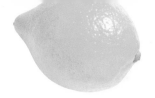

© Element/HarperCollins*Publishers* 2002

First published in Great Britain in 1997
by ELEMENT BOOKS LIMITED

Reprinted 1998, March, July 1999

This edition published in 2002
by Element, an Imprint of
HarperCollins*Publishers*,
77-85 Fulham Palace Road,
Hammersmith, London W6 8JB

NOTE FROM THE PUBLISHER
Any information given in this book is not
intended to be taken as a replacement for
medical advice. Any person with a
condition requiring medical attention
should consult a qualified practitioner or
therapist.

Designed and created with
The Bridgewater Book Company Ltd

THE BRIDGEWATER BOOK COMPANY LTD
Art Director Kevin Knight
Designers Andrew Milne, Jane Lanaway
Page layout Chris Lanaway
Managing Editor Anne Townley
Project co-ordinator Fiona Corbridge
Picture Research Lynda Marshall
Three dimensional models
Mark Jamieson
Photography Ian Parsons, Guy Ryecart
Illustrations Andrew Milne,
Pip Adams
Medical Illustrations
Michael Courtney

Editorial consultants
BOOK CREATION SERVICES LTD
Series Editor Karen Sullivan

Printed and bound by Printing Express,
Hong Kong

British Library Cataloguing in
Publication data available

Library of Congress Cataloging in
Publication data available

ISBN 0-00-714039-8

The publishers wish to thank the following for the
use of pictures: Bridgeman Art Library and e.t.
archive

Special thanks go to:
Natalie Gray, Julia Holden, Claire Morgan
and Neil Redfern, Stephen Sparshatt and
Carys Lecrass, Yvonne Worth.

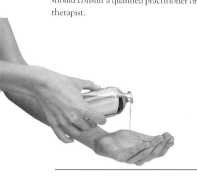

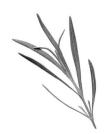

Contents

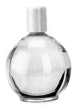

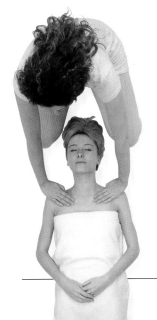

What is massage?

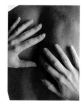

ABOVE **The power of touch: therapy since ancient times.**

MASSAGE IS ONE of the oldest, simplest forms of therapy and is a system of stroking, pressing, and kneading different areas of the body to relieve pain, relax, stimulate, and tone the body. Massage does much more than create a pleasant sensation on the skin, it also works on the soft tissues (the muscles, tendons, and ligaments) to improve muscle tone. Although it largely affects those muscles just under the skin, its benefits may also reach the deeper layers of muscle and possibly even the organs themselves. Massage also stimulates blood circulation and assists the lymphatic system (which runs parallel to the circulatory system), improving the elimination of waste throughout the body.

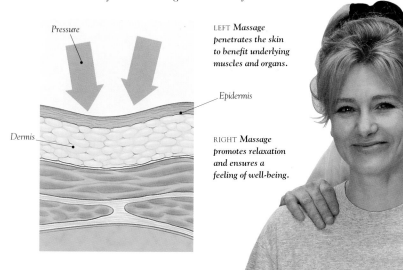

Pressure

Epidermis

Dermis

LEFT **Massage penetrates the skin to benefit underlying muscles and organs.**

RIGHT **Massage promotes relaxation and ensures a feeling of well-being.**

THE EFFECTS OF MASSAGE

Although a single massage will be enjoyable, the effects of massage are cumulative and a course of massage treatments will bring the most benefits. Regular massage can have the effect of strengthening and toning the entire body mechanism, and so help to prevent unnecessary strains and injuries that might otherwise occur due to excess tension and any resulting structural weaknesses. Massage can stimulate or calm the nervous system – depending upon what is required by the individual – and thus help reduce fatigue, leaving the receiver with a feeling of replenished energy. At its best, massage has the potential to restore the individual physically, mentally, and spiritually.

SOME BENEFITS OF MASSAGE

- relaxing
- soothing
- healing
- reassuring
- eases tension, stiffness, and pain
- improves breathing
- improves circulation
- enhances well-being

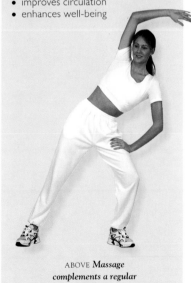

ABOVE *Massage complements a regular exercise program.*

A short history

MASSAGE HAS been used in Eastern healing disciplines for thousands of years. There is evidence in the form of wall paintings, tomb art, ceramics, woodcuts, and illustrations, of massage techniques being used in China, Japan, Egypt, and Persia as long ago as 5,000 years. In the West, massage was certainly used in Greek and Roman medicine – even Hippocrates, the "father of medicine," is said to have recommended "rubbing" to aid the

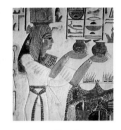

ABOVE *Egyptian art depicting oil jars used during massage.*

body. The clinical use of massage disappeared during the Middle Ages and was not revived until the 16th century, when French surgeon Ambroise Paré encouraged its practice once more.

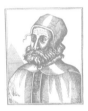

ABOVE **Ambroise Paré preached the virtues of massage.**

RIGHT **Massage therapies span the world.**

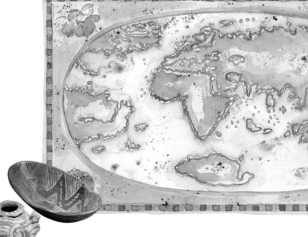

In the early 19th century Per Henrik Ling, a Swedish writer and fencing master, became famous for developing a comprehensive system of gymnastics and massage, and in 1813 a school was established in Stockholm which was the first to offer courses in massage as part of its program. Ling's massage techniques are at the root of many of the massage systems in existence today.

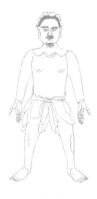

LEFT *Hippocrates and Galen: famous physicians in ancient Greece.*

DIFFERENT TYPES OF MASSAGE AND MASSAGE-RELATED THERAPIES

•

Acupressure
(Oriental pressure therapy)

•

Aromatherapy
(plant essence therapy)

•

Naturopathy
(a system adopting different methods to help the body heal itself)

•

Reflexology
(pressure therapy on reflex zones on the feet)

•

Rolfing
(very deep tissue massage therapy)

•

Shiatsu
(Oriental massage therapy)

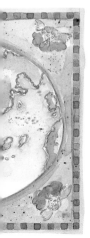

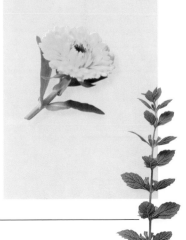

ABOVE *The Chinese people's use of massage dates back about 5,000 years.*

Setting the scene

TOWELS AND OIL

ENVIRONMENT

It is essential to create a warm, comfortable environment for your partner or client.

• Use soft lighting for a more relaxing atmosphere.

• Warm the room beforehand to ensure your partner or client doesn't get cold.

• Select a time when you won't be interrupted.

• Wear loose, comfortable clothing.

• Make sure you have clean hands and short nails.

• Remove jewelry from your hands and wrists.

• If you have long hair, it is best to tie or clip it back.

• Should you wish to play music, choose something soothing.

Aim to complete a full-body massage in one to one-and-a-quarter hours. If you continue for much longer than this you risk tiring yourself, and your partner or client may start to feel chilly and uncomfortable.

LEFT *Making initial contact with the client.*

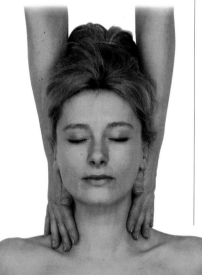

STARTING OFF

Begin the massage by placing your hands gently on the receiver's shoulders to make an initial, gentle contact. Breathe in and then out, and focus your attention on your hands and the natural healing energy flowing through your body.

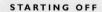

EQUIPMENT

Y ou will need a firm, padded surface on which to work. This can be a massage table, or a small cotton or foam mattress placed on the floor.

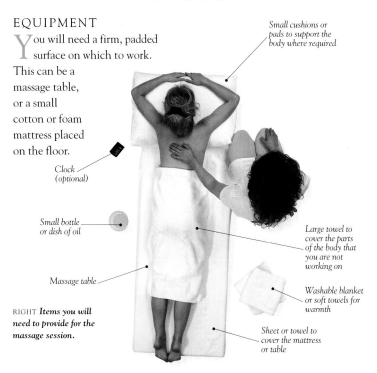

Small cushions or pads to support the body where required

Clock (optional)

Small bottle or dish of oil

Massage table

Large towel to cover the parts of the body that you are not working on

Washable blanket or soft towels for warmth

Sheet or towel to cover the mattress or table

RIGHT **Items you will need to provide for the massage session.**

MASSAGE OILS

Try different oils to see which ones suit you best. Here are some commonly used types:

- mineral (including baby oil)
- soya
- peach or apricot kernel
- grapeseed
- sunflower
- almond (expensive)
- olive oil (very sticky)
- peanut oil

Use only enough oil to cover the particular area you are working on with a thin film of oil. Using too much oil makes the body slippery and difficult to work on.

LEFT **A selection of massage oils.**

Professional treatment

MASSAGE IS *a simple, safe form of therapy, but there are situations where it should be avoided. Before you start, check the list of contraindications on page 50. If you are unsure about whether it is safe to undergo massage, consult your physician first.*

SEEKING PROFESSIONAL TREATMENT

There are various reasons to seek treatment from a professional. These include:
- stiffness, headaches, muscle pain, or discomfort
- stress-related disorders
- as a complement to an exercise program
- to enhance general well-being
- as a delicious treat
- recommendation from another practitioner as part of a treatment process

WHAT TO EXPECT FROM A PROFESSIONAL TREATMENT

Massage treatments will vary, but in general the process is as follows.

The therapist will first take a case history and ask you about:
• Your medical history (previous accidents, injuries, broken bones, operations, major illnesses, allergies, pregnancies, menstrual problems, or whether you are taking any medication or having any other treatment).

LEFT *The process of massage is a partnership between client and therapist.*

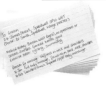

ABOVE *The therapist will take notes.*

• Your lifestyle (occupation, exercise, diet, sleeping habits).
• Whether you have any back trouble, headaches, or are under stress.
• If there is any particular area of the body that you would like worked on.

You will be asked to undress and lie, covered with a towel, on the massage table. Treatment lasts about an hour. Relax, enjoy the massage, and simply concentrate on your breathing. At the end of the treatment you will be covered with a blanket and asked to rest for a minute or two before getting up.

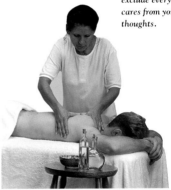

LEFT *Relax and enjoy the massage: try to exclude everyday cares from your thoughts.*

MASSAGE IN COMBINATION WITH OTHER THERAPIES

In most cases a course of massage treatment may be safely undertaken either on its own, in combination with other forms of treatment, or as part of a normal, healthy way of life.

Practitioners, osteopaths, chiropractics, acupuncturists, reflexologists, personal trainers, dance and yoga teachers may often recommend massage, but there are occasions when it might not be suitable. Homeopathic remedies, for example, may need to be taken in isolation in order for the homeopath to effectively monitor the results of prescribed remedies. If you are already undergoing any form of treatment, always check with your practitioner beforehand. If you experiment with different therapies, leave time between them.

RIGHT *It is best to leave at least 48 hours between treatments.*

Monday 15 June
Reflexology - Jenny Wood 3 p.m

Tuesday 16 June

Wednesday 17 June
Acupuncture - John Gray 11 a.m

Thursday 18 June

Friday 19 June
Massage - Joanna Simon 2 p.m

Saturday 20 June

Sunday 21 June

The importance of touch

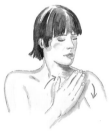

ABOVE *The healing touch: soothe tension, aches and pains.*

TOUCH HAS *always been our instinctive reaction to pain, discomfort, and sorrow – in ourselves and in those around us. We automatically "rub better" any bumps, bruises, aches, and pains, hold the hand of someone in crisis, and give a reassuring hug to anyone who is upset. Touch is possibly the oldest method of any type of healing and from this simple art have grown such powerful disciplines as laying-on of hands, osteopathy, chiropractic, shiatsu, reflexology, and, of course, massage.*

ABOVE *Touch is a fundamental bond between parent and child.*

A LOVING TOUCH

The way we use our hands in massage is of vital importance: a true sensitivity, a caring attitude and faith in our own ability to help can have the most profound effect, bringing about a sense of pleasure and wholeness in the person receiving the massage.

AN ESSENTIAL INGREDIENT

Touch is an essential ingredient to our overall well-being. From infancy, cuddles and caresses are a basic source of emotional nourishment, making us feel loved and wanted and helping us develop a healthy, strong self-image. Throughout our lives, this physical contact continues to be an important factor in our well-being.

Techniques

DIFFERENT TYPES OF STROKE AND PRESSURE

There are a variety of different strokes that can be used, ranging from the most delicate touch with the fingertips to focused deep-tissue work. All strokes can be varied in speed and pressure. Keeping your hands relaxed, begin working slowly and rhythmically, gradually building up speed and pressure as you experiment.

Some basic points

• As a general rule, strokes should be made firmly in the direction of the heart, and then lightly for the return stroke.
• By varying their intensity, strokes can be used either to stimulate or relax.
• Ideally the receiver should experience the massage as one long series of rhythmic strokes.

LEFT **Firm outward strokes; lighter return strokes.**

PRACTICE

Begin by practicing on yourself. Use your own leg to try out the different strokes. Once you are familiar with these, feel free to improvize and adapt the strokes you have learnt, or even invent new ones. These can be allowed to develop as you work.

MASSAGE POSITION

Avoid working only from your hands and shoulders. Use the weight and movement of your whole body to improve the fluidity of your strokes and to help you when you wish to use more pressure.

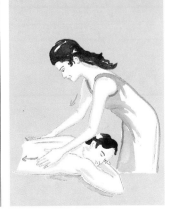

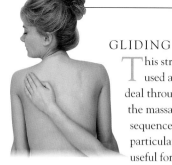

ABOVE *The gliding stroke can be light or firm.*

GLIDING

This stroke is used a great deal throughout the massage sequence and is particularly useful for applying oil to the body. It can be a feather-light or a firm, reassuring stroke. Keeping the fingers together and hands outstretched, glide the hands forward along the length of the body or limb, retaining contact with the flat of the hand. The strokes you employ can be either long or circular, using one or both hands. The function of gliding strokes is to relax and stretch your patient's muscles.

KNEADING

Kneading is a firm stroke used on a specific area to help release muscle tension and improve circulation.

Gently grasp the area (e.g. calf, thigh, or fleshy area over the hip) with both hands and make a kneading action similar to that of kneading dough.

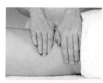

LEFT *The firm kneading stroke.*

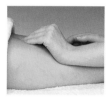

LEFT *Draining a large area such as the thigh.*

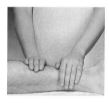

LEFT *Draining a small area such as the calf.*

DRAINING

A light- to mid-pressure stroke which relaxes and stretches the muscles and improves the circulation. Use either the heel of the hand on larger areas (e.g. thigh) or the thumbs on smaller areas (e.g. calves, forearms). With one hand following the other, push firmly using the heel or thumb of first one hand and then the next, traveling slowly upward along the limb or muscle.

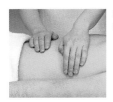

LEFT *The pulling stroke.*

Start with hands placed either side of the body or limb. Moving the hands in a forward and back motion across the body, progress slowly up toward the head.

PULLING

This stroke can be used to pull and stretch the muscles of the trunk, and the legs. Use alternating hands in a pulling motion, gradually moving them up the body.

WRINGING

This stroke is similar to "pulling", but works right across the body or limb. This is a good stroke with which to finish a particular sequence and can be used on the torso, legs, and arms.

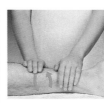

LEFT *Continuing the wringing stroke up the limb.*

FRICTION STROKES

These are deeper strokes which allow you to work around joints and into the muscles and tendons, to iron out knots and release tension. Using the thumbs or fingertips, work slowly and firmly into the area, making tiny circular movements. Different individuals will prefer different pressures – some will only be able to tolerate light pressure, others will want you to work as deeply as possible.

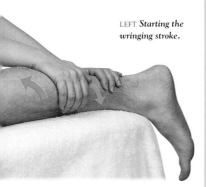

LEFT *Starting the wringing stroke.*

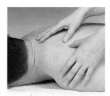

LEFT *Friction strokes: making tiny circular movements with the thumbs.*

PERCUSSIVE STROKES

Percussive strokes, such as hacking, cupping, and plucking, are used to stimulate areas, improve circulation, and release muscle tension. They can be used on the shoulders, arms, legs, buttocks, and gently along the back. Do not use percussive strokes directly on the spine. These strokes are not an essential part of any massage sequence, but you may wish to incorporate some of them into your routine. They can be performed very lightly, or with more intensity, as appropriate. Remember to keep your hands and wrists as relaxed as possible.

ABOVE *A variation on hacking: pummeling.*

motion up and down the body. As a variation on this stroke, curl the fingers into loose fists to create more of a pummeling effect on the body.

HACKING

With hands open and palms facing each other, make an alternating "chopping"

CUPPING

Cup hands and face palms downward. Keeping hands cupped, gently beat up and down along the body.

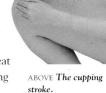

ABOVE *The cupping stroke.*

PINCHING OR PLUCKING

Gently lift small amounts of flesh or muscle and let it slide through the fingers.

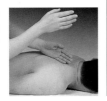

RIGHT *The hacking stroke.*

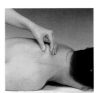

LEFT *Pinching a small roll of flesh.*

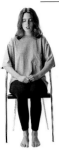

The art of massage

ATTITUDE AND INTENTION *are of primary importance – always begin a massage in a positive, caring frame of mind. Take time to relax and center yourself before you start the massage session.*

Try these techniques to focus and prepare yourself.
- Close your eyes and sit quietly for a few minutes.
- Concentrate on your breathing.
- Let go of any thoughts that may be worrying you or are cluttering your mind.
- Imagine all unnecessary tension flowing out of you each time you exhale.

A final preparation
Spend two minutes "warming up" your hands before you start.
- Shake hands loosely from the wrist to get rid of residual tension.
- Flex, stretch, and curl fingers to loosen the muscles.
- Gently massage each hand (almost as if you were putting on some hand cream).

ESSENTIAL OILS

OILING
- Be sparing with the amount of oil you use.
- Place ½ teaspoon (5ml) of oil in the palm of your hand and rub hands gently together.
- Using a gliding stroke, cover the part of the body that you want to work on first with a thin film of oil.
- If you wish, add a couple of drops of your favorite essential oil (for example, lavender can be relaxing or invigorating, rosemary is stimulating, Roman chamomile is soothing).
- Keep the oil close to you in a small bottle or dish.
- Do not pour the oil into your hand directly above your client, in case it drips accidentally.

POURING OUT OIL

ABOVE AND RIGHT
Keep the oil handy in a bottle or dish.

Back

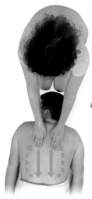

ABOVE *Beginning the back massage.*

DURING A *full-body massage the largest amount of time is usually devoted to the back and shoulders, partly because the back represents such a large part of the body, and partly because this is a very common place for people to accumulate tension.*

1 Position yourself at your partner's head with them lying on their front, face downward or turned to one side, and arms by their sides. Starting on their upper back, glide hands slowly down either side of the spine, back up the sides of the body, and lightly over the shoulders.

> **TIP**
>
> Avoid rough or sudden movements as you cover and uncover the different areas of the body. Make sure you place the towel gently and avoid abrupt movements that might be disturbing to someone in a relaxed state.

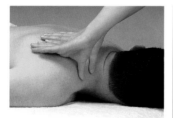

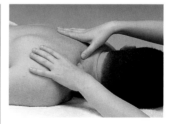

2 Turn your partner's head gently to their right and work on their left shoulder. Using both hands, starting at the base of the neck, make firm strokes outward along the shoulder and off at the top of the arm.

3 Use the thumbs to work into the muscles at the base of the neck. Pay particular attention to any knots or areas of tightness that you find here, working firmly and slowly into the muscles, making tiny circles.

UPPER BACK

1 Move to the right of your partner. Grasp the top of their right shoulder with your right hand and place your left hand on their lower back. Draw the left hand firmly up along the side of the spine and the right hand down to meet it. Continue the stroke, moving both hands upward over the shoulder.

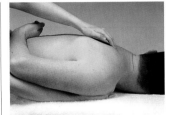

2 Slide hands down the arm and, taking the elbow in your right hand and the hand in your left, lift the arm and place it behind the back.

3 Cupping your right hand under the right shoulder, use the thumb or fingers of your left hand to work from the shoulder down around the shoulderblade. Stroke upward and over the whole shoulderblade. Use the fingers and thumb to stroke firmly along the protruding bone of the top of the shoulderblade. Move the arm back to its original position and turn your partner's head to the other side. Repeat the above sequence for the other side of the body.

LEFT *Beginning the upper back sequence.*

> **TIP**
>
> Always avoid working directly over the spine, unless you are using extremely gentle, or feathering-type strokes. Work into the muscles either side of the spine instead.

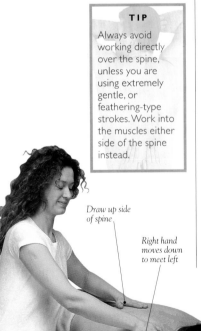

Draw up side of spine

Right hand moves down to meet left

LOWER BACK

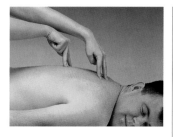

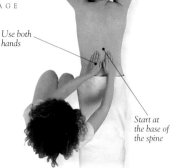

Use both hands

Start at the base of the spine

1 Position yourself next to your partner's lower back. Placing the first and index fingers of each hand on either side of the spine, with one hand slightly behind the other, make rhythmic, overlapping movements all the way down the back.

2 Oil the lower back, starting at the base of the spine (the sacrum) gliding up, on either side of the spine to the ribcage, and down the sides of the body, returning to the starting position.

3 Using a friction stroke with the thumbs, make small overlapping circles over the sacrum, gradually moving up the sides of the spine to the ribcage.

LEFT **Using a friction stroke to make small circles.**

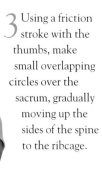

Use your thumbs

Move up each side of the spine

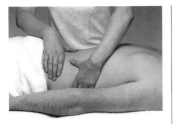

ABOVE *Knead the whole hip area.*

BELOW *Finish by stroking down the whole length of the spine.*

TIP

When performed in a slow, focused way, the massage sequence can invoke an almost meditative state in the client, and perhaps even in the masseur too!

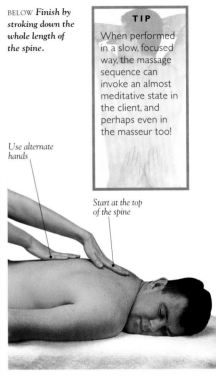

Use alternate hands

Start at the top of the spine

4 Shift your position slightly so that you are facing your partner and begin working on the opposite side of the body. Make big gliding circles moving up the side of the spine, around the ribcage, down the side of the body, over the fleshy part of the hip, and back to the starting position. Using firm generous kneading strokes, work gradually over the entire hip area.

TIP

For comfort you may wish to place a small cushion under the upper chest, under the ankles, and under the ribcage, just below the breasts (for women).

FEEDBACK

Ask for some feedback, but it's preferable to discuss the patient's likes and dislikes more fully at the end of the session.

5 Place hands, facing across the body, with one on each hip, and use a wringing stroke all the way up the body to the shoulders. Changing position, repeat the above sequence for the opposite side of the body. To finish the sequence, stroke down the whole length of the spine several times using alternate hands.

Neck and shoulders

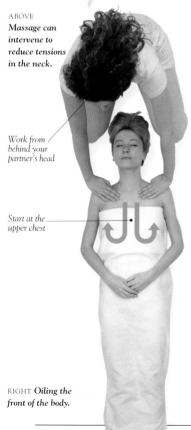

FOR MANY *people, the neck and shoulders are common areas of soreness and tension. Working at a desk or a computer all day helps to create such problems. To have this pain eased away can be a source of great pleasure.*

ABOVE
Massage can intervene to reduce tensions in the neck.

Work from behind your partner's head

Start at the upper chest

RIGHT **Oiling the front of the body.**

EMOTIONAL RELEASE

Massage can sometimes trigger an emotional reaction – anything from tears to uncontrollable laughter. If this happens, just recognize it as an emotional release and continue with the massage using soothing, gentle strokes, until the receiver is calm once more.

1 Position yourself at your partner's head, with them lying on their back. Oil the front of the body, starting with hands on their upper chest, then move down over the breastbone, out around the ribcage, and back up the sides of the body to the starting position. Place hands on upper chest, fingers pointing toward each other and press down, gliding the hands out toward the top of the arm.

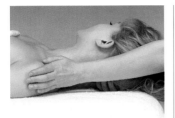

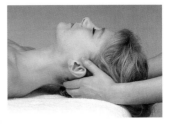

2 Cradle the head in one hand and turn it slightly toward the right. With the other hand, glide firmly out from the center of the chest to the top of the arm, back along the top of the shoulder, and up the back of the neck to the base of the skull.

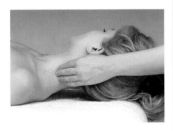

3 Make little circles along the back of the neck to release tension, then continue back down the side of the neck to the chest. Stroke firmly down the side of the neck and out along the top of the shoulder, stretching the neck muscles.

4 Turn the head back to the center with both hands supporting the head under the neck, and pull gently to stretch out the neck muscles.

5 Turn the head to the opposite side and repeat the sequence for the other shoulder. Return the head to the center and pull gently. Make small, overlapping, circular movements up the back of the neck to the skull and then stroke up the back of the head and off. Gently lower the head.

BELOW *Turn the head to the opposite side and repeat the sequence.*

Make smooth movements

Gently turn the head

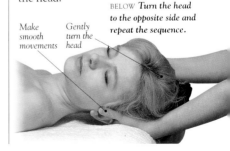

Chest

AS YOU WORK *around the body, change your position so that you are comfortable. Involve your whole body – whether standing or sitting, use the floor as a lever to help you and let your body move in the same rhythm as the strokes you are creating.*

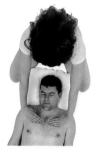
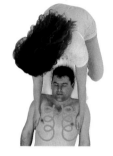
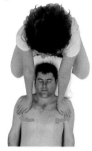

1 Using the fingertips, work in between the upper ribs, stroking from the center of the chest outward. Repeat three or four times, moving down to the next rib with each repeat.

2 Using small overlapping circles, massage down over the breastbone and sweep down over the ribcage and back up the sides of the body.

4 To finish, place both hands on upper chest, pointing outward toward the shoulders, and pressing a little, glide hands firmly out and off the shoulders.

3 Starting at the bottom of the ribcage, use a pulling motion up each side of the body. Repeat on the other side.

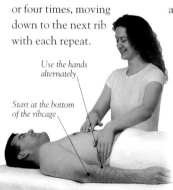

Use the hands alternately

Start at the bottom of the ribcage

LEFT **Make a pulling stroke on the side of the body. Both hands are used alternately.**

26

Abdomen

THE ABDOMEN *is the softest, least-protected area of the body and is, therefore, an area of great vulnerability for many people. Always work very gently and rhythmically in this area, only increasing the pressure once the receiver feels secure and relaxed.*

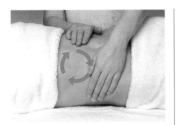

1 Oil in large circles working around the navel in a clockwise direction, using both hands.

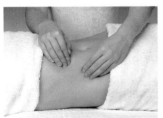

2 Continue circling the abdomen and begin to work a little more firmly using the fingertips to make small circles.

3 Place one hand either side of the body, on each hip, and wring up the body in a forward and backward motion. Then stroke up over the ribcage, over the breastbone and off at the shoulders.

TIP

Some people may not like you to touch their abdomen. When you reach this point in the sequence, you might like to first check with your partner that they feel comfortable with you massaging the stomach area.

RIGHT **Wring up the body, moving the hands backward and forward.**

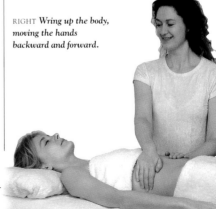

Face and head

A FACE MASSAGE *and head massage is a particularly pleasurable experience – most people will be surprised at the amount of tension they hold here, particularly around the jaw. There is not usually time for a full face and head massage as part of a full-body massage. You might like to try it on its own or in combination with a back and shoulder massage.*

FACE

1 Cup hands around the head, with thumbs resting on the forehead and fingertips at the temples. Smooth out the forehead in strips – starting along the eyebrows, working up toward the hairline.

Thumbs on forehead

Fingertips at temples

The throat is another vulnerable area of the body. Although the sides and back of the neck can be massaged, avoid working directly across the throat itself.

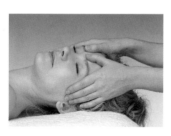

2 Press between the eyebrows with your thumbs. Repeat, moving up the center of the forehead to the hairline.

LEFT *Cup the hands
and rest them on the
head, with the thumbs
at the forehead.*

*Place hands
gently on head*

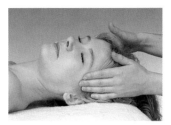

3 Massage temples, using
circular motion with fingers.
Continue circles down along the
jawbone to the chin.

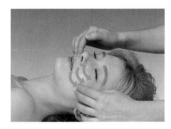

4 Using your fingertips, draw a
line under the cheekbone
and out to the temples. Repeat,
taking the line lower down the
cheek each time.

SKIN TEXTURE

The face is naturally more oily
than the other parts of the body.
Unless the receiver has
particularly dry skin, you will
not need to add extra oil at
this stage.

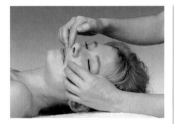

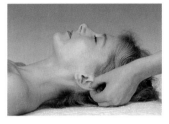

5 Use the fingertips to "draw" a big moustache shape from the upper lip out to the temples, and circle the temples one more time.

7 Gently massage the ears between your thumbs and fingers, starting at the earlobe and moving around and up to the top of the ear.

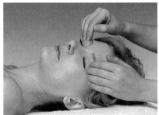

8 Pull ears very gently, again starting with the lobe and moving gradually to the top of the ear.

6 Press softly around the upper bone of the eye sockets, starting from the bridge of the nose, out to the corner of the eye. Repeat, this time working carefully around the eye socket under the eyes.

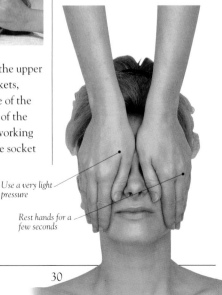

Use a very light pressure

RIGHT **Warn your partner before cupping your hands over their eyes.**

Rest hands for a few seconds

9 Cup hands and rest them over the eyes (it's best to warn your partner before you do this). Ask your partner to breathe in and out deeply several times. Release the hands.

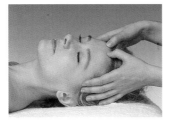

HEAD

1 Cup forehead in hands once more and press in the middle of the forehead at hairline. Continue pressing upward to the crown of the head.

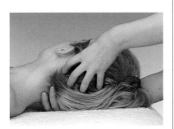

2 Supporting the head in the hands and with fingers at the base of the skull, massage the entire scalp.

3 Draw fingers lightly through the hair several times, and off at the crown.

TIP

If your partner's hair is very thick, avoid the possibility of getting your fingers caught in tangles by drawing your fingers over the top of the hair instead.

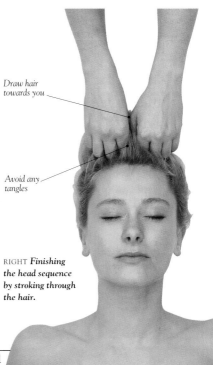

Draw hair towards you

Avoid any tangles

RIGHT *Finishing the head sequence by stroking through the hair.*

Arms and hands

OUR ARMS and hands are used constantly throughout the day, and are required for our greatest expressions of emotion – from angry outbursts to tender caresses. An arm and hand massage can release tension and relax us, improving our sense of well-being.

ABOVE **Flexing the arm muscles.**

ARMS

> **TIP**
>
> While working on the limbs, make sure they are as relaxed as possible. If you notice that your partner is "holding on," ask them gently to let the limb go.

1 Starting at the wrist, oil the arm and top of the shoulder, making contact with the whole of the arm. Sandwich the shoulder between both hands and glide hands outward and down the arm.

RIGHT **Working on the forearm. Hold the arm with one hand and work with the other.**

2 Lift the forearm with one hand. With the other, drain from the wrist up along the forearm.

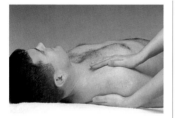

It may be more comfortable to sit by your partner

Drain the forearm towards the elbow

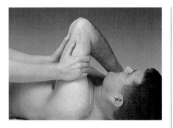

3 Lift the whole of the arm and, keeping the upper arm at a right angle to the body, let the hand flop. Grasp the elbow with hands and squeeze downward along the upper arm toward the shoulder joint (rather like squeezing toothpaste). Place arm back at the side of the body.

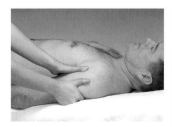

4 Starting at the top of the arm squeeze gently between the hands, making a spreading motion with the flattened thumbs. Continue down the arm to the wrist, pausing at the elbow to work into the joint, using friction strokes.

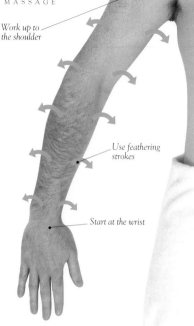

Work up to the shoulder

Use feathering strokes

Start at the wrist

ABOVE **Use both hands to wring up the arm.**

5 Using both hands, wring up the arm, starting at the wrist and working all the way up to the shoulder.

6 Stroke the arm from the shoulder down to the hand using light, feathering strokes.

7 Remain in position to finish the sequence by working on your partner's hand.

HANDS

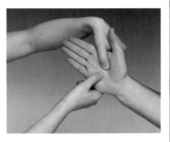

1 Sandwich your partner's hand between your own for a few seconds. Using your thumbs, massage the palm of the hand.

2 Massage the back of the hand, working in between the bones to help release any tension. Do not press too hard.

3 Massage each of the fingers and the thumb in turn, squeezing, rotating, and pulling them gently.

BELOW *Massaging the back of the hand, working between the bones.*

> **TIP**
>
> Find a comfortable position for working on your partner's hand. You may find it best to rest the hand on your leg, if you are seated alongside.

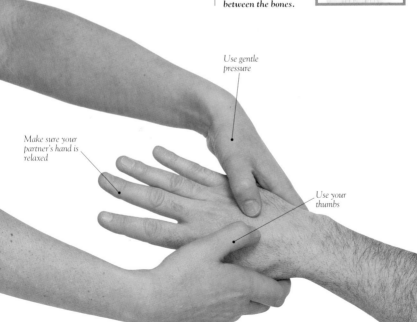

Use gentle pressure

Make sure your partner's hand is relaxed

Use your thumbs

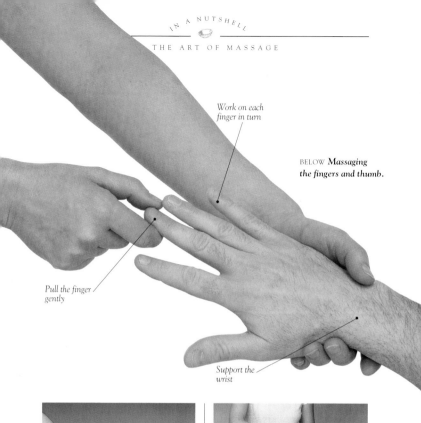

Work on each finger in turn

BELOW **Massaging the fingers and thumb.**

Pull the finger gently

Support the wrist

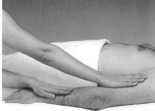

4 Using light strokes, draw your hands down your partner's arm, down the hand, and off at the fingertips. This finishes the hand massage.

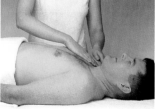

5 Move round to the opposite side of your partner. Now repeat every stage of the arm and hand sequence for this side of the body.

Legs and feet

ALL TOO OFTEN *we take our bodies for granted,*
putting continual demands on ourselves. Our legs
and feet frequently get ignored and small twinges
and discomforts go unheeded. Massage provides
the means to ease these tensions and revitalize this
weight-bearing part of the body. People whose
jobs entail a lot of standing will find a leg and foot
massage especially useful. Like the arms, the legs
are also worked on individually.

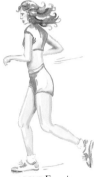

ABOVE **Exercise**
places extra
demands on the
hands and feet.

LEGS

1 Oil the entire leg, beginning
at the ankle, working
up and over the hip,
back down the leg
and over the feet.
Drain up from the
ankle using the
thumbs, stroke gently over the
back of the knee, and, using the
heels of the hands, continue
draining the thigh up to the
hip joint. Glide hands
back down to the ankles
and off over the feet.

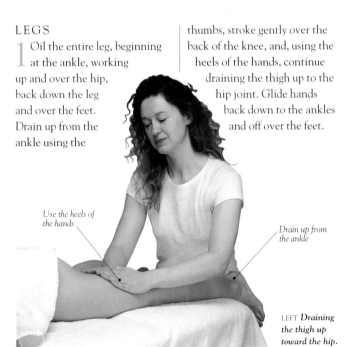

Use the heels of
the hands

Drain up from
the ankle

LEFT **Draining**
the thigh up
toward the hip.

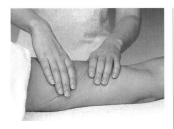

TIP

If the person you are massaging has hairy legs or chest, you will need to use more oil as hair tends to absorb the oil more quickly.

2 Knead the calves and the thighs, gently stroking over the back of the knee as you move from one leg to the other.

CAUTION

The calves can be tender, particularly if your partner does a lot of exercise, such as running or cycling.

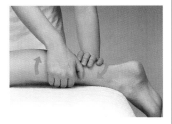

3 Wring up the legs from ankle to buttock, again being careful not to put any pressure on the back of the knee area.

4 Complete the sequence by using light, feathering strokes all the way down the leg.

FEET

1 Foot massage can be both soothing and invigorating, and even people with ticklish feet respond to firm strokes. Bend the leg at the knee and work the ankle joint around, using a circling motion.

BELOW *Bend the leg up, grasp the foot, and gently work the ankle joint.*

Rotate the foot

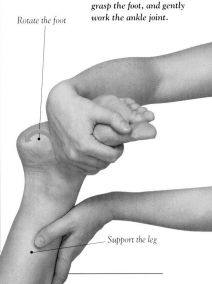

Support the leg

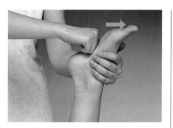

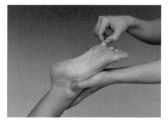

2 Hold the foot firmly in one hand and use the palm of the other to stroke along the foot from heel to toes. Make the hand into a fist and, with the finger joints pressed into the foot, stroke firmly along sole of the foot. Squeeze the heel.

3 Holding the foot in both hands, work along the sole of the foot, making small overlapping circles with the thumbs.

4 Work between the tendons on the front of the foot, all the way down to the toes. Massage each of the toes, squeezing and gently pulling each one in turn.

5 Massage the foot between the heels of both hands, using a circular motion. Stroke firmly along the sole of the foot and lower the leg. Repeat for the other leg.

Use your thumbs

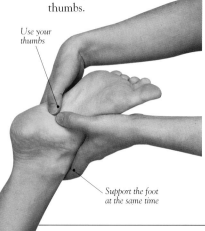

Support the foot at the same time

TIP

If your partner turns out to have ticklish feet, try increasing the pressure of the strokes you use.

LEFT *Working along the sole of the foot, making overlapping circles.*

FRONT OF LEGS

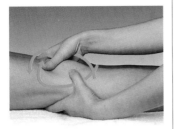

1 Oil up the entire leg. Drain up from the calf to the knee using the thumbs. Holding the back of the knee with your left hand, stroke with your right hand in a clockwise direction up around the knee cap and round to the back of the knee; then stroke with the left hand in an anticlockwise direction. Repeat this sequence several times.

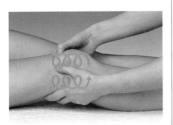

2 Work into the area directly around the knee cap. Use your thumbs to make small, overlapping circles.

3 Drain up from the knee cap to the top of the thigh, using the heels of the hands. Glide hands back down to the ankle. Wring all the way up the leg, starting at the ankle, and then knead the thigh area. Use light feathering strokes down the length of the leg and over the feet to finish the front of the leg. Repeat on the other leg.

END OF SESSION

Finish each massage with long connecting strokes starting at the forehead, over the top of the head to the base of the skull, along the shoulders and down the hands and then, starting at the forehead once more, over the top of the head to the base of the skull, then down the front of the body, and down the legs.

It is also a good idea to use this procedure on yourself to "close down" after completing a massage.

LEFT *Long, connecting strokes denote the end of the massage.*

Babies and children

BABIES AND CHILDREN *usually enjoy being massaged as much as adults, but will often only keep still for a short space of time. The strokes you have learned can be used on babies and children – just adapt them to allow for their size and the fact that their little bodies will not have built up the same chronic tensions that adults can suffer from. Just explore and discover what your child likes best.*

LITTLE HELPERS

Children will love to try some massage for themselves. The delicate stroke of a child on the head and down the back can be immensely soothing. Children may even be happy to pound your tense shoulders for you, or walk up and down your back!

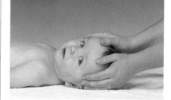

ABOVE *Stroking across the forehead.*

FRONT OF THE BODY

1 Starting with the child on their back, gently stroke their face, starting in the middle of the forehead and working out to the temples.

2 Stroke across the cheeks from nose to the ears and then from the cheeks down to the chin. Gently stroke across the eyebrows, and back around under the eye. Make gentle circles around the temples.

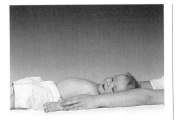

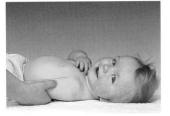

3 Stroke up the front of the body and out along the arms.

4 Make clockwise circles around the navel using both hands. Do gentle "wringing" strokes across the abdomen and up the body.

5 Lift arms one at a time and stroke the length of the arm from shoulder to the hand. Use one hand to squeeze the arm, starting from the shoulder and moving down the arm.

6 Massage the hand and squeeze and rotate each of the fingers in turn.

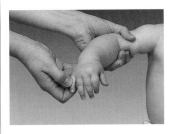

7 Repeat for the other arm. Gently drain up the leg. Wring or squeeze up the leg.

8 Stroke down the leg using a light, feathering stroke.

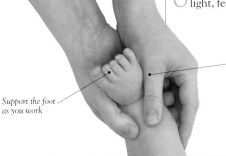

Use a light pressure

Support the foot as you work

LEFT **Working from the ankle, wring or squeeze up the leg.**

BACK OF THE BODY

1 Turn the child on to their front and gently stroke their back. Stroke up and over the back and along the arms.

2 Gently knead the child's shoulders.

3 Make a gentle wringing stroke up over the body. If your child is a baby, massage their rear using gentle kneading or pinching strokes.

MASSAGE STROKES

As a general rule, the strokes you use will need to be much lighter on children. The younger the child, the smaller and more delicate the strokes will need to be.

If the child you are working on is very young, then you can sit on the floor and massage him or her on your lap. Otherwise spread a towel on the floor or on any safe, raised surface.

Favorite toy

Knead shoulders

Massage rear

LEFT **Put the child on their front and begin massaging their back.**

4 Smooth down the spine using alternating hands, starting at the base of the neck and working down to the base of the spine. Use gliding strokes down the legs. Bend the knee up and work on the foot.

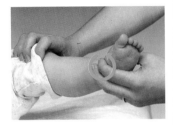

5 Work around the anklebone with your fingertips Sandwich foot between heels of hand and massage, moving both hands in a circular motion.

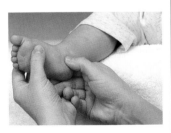

6 Gently squeeze the heel with one hand and massage up the sole of the child's foot using the thumbs of your other hand.

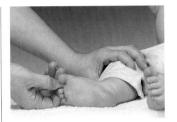

7 Massage the toes, gently squeezing, rotating and pulling each one in turn. Sandwich the foot between your hands and hold it firmly for a few seconds. Turn the baby over.

CAUTION

Be very gentle when working with babies and children. Do not pursue the session if the child begins to fidget.

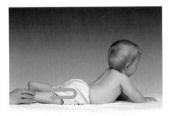

8 Stroke from one foot up the leg, across the sacrum (base of the spine), and back down the other leg. Use light strokes down the body, starting from the top of head right down to the feet.

Massage in pregnancy

MANY WOMEN SUFFER *from aches and pains, stiffness and tension during pregnancy. Gentle massage can often help to relieve problems such as backache,* sleeplessness, edema, headaches, *and other minor complaints.*

ABOVE **Lemon oil is ideal for massage.**

BEFORE BIRTH

Back pain is extremely common in pregnancy (as well as during the period of breastfeeding, or of having to carry small children). It can be relieved by massage to the whole of the back area, the neck, legs, and feet, and by gentle stroking of the abdomen. Poor circulation also affects many pregnant women, and can be helped by a general body massage, which stimulates and improves the blood flow throughout the body. Leg massage, stroking

from the ankles up toward the thighs, can help relax the body, relieve pain and reduce swelling in the legs (but avoid working directly over varicose veins). For women who develop problems sleeping, the soothing effects of massage can help relax and calm. Some pregnant women claim

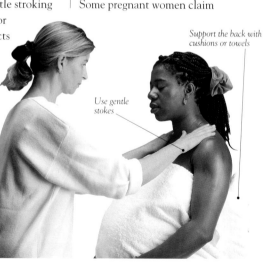

Support the back with cushions or towels

Use gentle stokes

RIGHT **Massage to the shoulders and arms can reduce tension.**

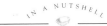
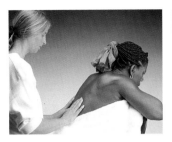

ABOVE *A pregnant woman can sit astride a chair for a back massage.*

WHEN AND HOW TO MASSAGE

Although some schools recommend avoiding massage during the first three months of pregnancy, many women find gentle massage throughout their pregnancy to be very beneficial. When massaging a pregnant woman you must be very gentle, particularly on the abdomen and lower back. Avoid using deep pressure and percussive strokes (see page 18).

that lightly massaging the abdomen can even help to send the fetus to sleep.

As well as relaxing and soothing away physical symptoms, massage can be a wonderful way of including your partner and children in the course of your pregnancy.

Pregnant women should check with their physician before having a massage. In cases where the physician recommends that the lower back and abdomen area should be avoided, massage the face, hands, arms, and feet to assist in relaxation.

AROMATHERAPY OILS

You may add a few drops of essential oil to the carrier oil. Oils for use during pregnancy are:

- Mandarin
- Neroli
- Petitgrain
- Tangerine
- Ylang-ylang
- Geranium
- Lemon
- Sandalwood
- Tea tree

Oils which are not suitable for use in pregnancy are:

- Aniseed
- Arnica
- Basil
- Clary sage
- Cypress
- Fennel
- Jasmine
- Juniper
- Marjoram

Massage and movement

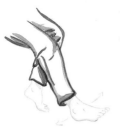

ABOVE *Suggest to your patient that simple swinging movements can aid mobility.*

USING PASSIVE *movements can be an extremely effective way of releasing tension in the joints and limbs. It is very rewarding but can be hard work – relaxed limbs are often much heavier than you would expect.*

NECK

1 Lie your partner on their back, and lift the head with both hands – keep lifting as far as is comfortable to stretch the back of the neck. Lower head slowly, pulling head gently to stretch the muscles at the back of the neck.

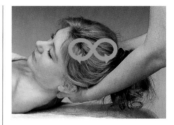

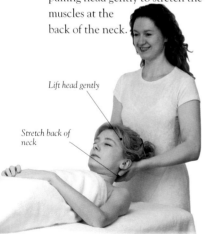

Lift head gently

Stretch back of neck

2 Hold the head in both hands, move it slowly from side to side, stretching the neck. Then draw a slow figure-eight shape with the head.

LEFT **Lifting the head to give a small stretch to the back of the neck.**

MOVEMENT STRETCHES

These stretches can be done as a separate sequence, or incorporated into a massage. The only exception are the leg rotations, which would usually only be done when your partner was clothed.

ARMS

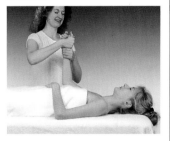

1 Lift the arm, asking your partner to relax and let you do the lifting (they may find this difficult). Holding your partner's hand securely, shake the arm, making sure the elbow is loose.

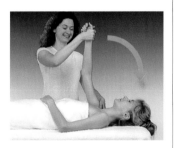

2 Straighten the arm and stretch it toward the ceiling. Keeping it straight, stretch it down on to the massage table above the head, to open out the shoulder joint. Raise the arm back to the ceiling and replace it at the side of the body.

HANDS

1 Lift the arm at the wrist, leaving the resting elbow on the massage table. Making sure arm and hand are completely relaxed, hold wrist firmly with both hands and shake the hand. Flex the wrist back and then stretch it forward.

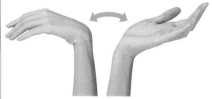

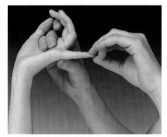

2 Supporting the back of the hand along the knuckles, flex the fingers back and then curl them forward. Rotate each finger individually at the knuckle joint and pull gently. Flex each finger gently backward and then curl it forward.

LEGS

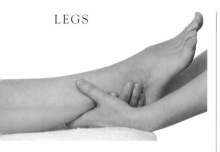

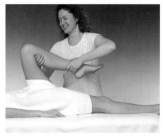

1 (Leg rotations are usually only done when the patient is clothed.) With your partner lying on their back, stretch each leg in turn by grasping the ankle with both hands and pulling the foot. This will stretch the leg muscles and help to release the hip joint.

3 Press your partner's knee gently down toward the chest, as far as is comfortable for them. This gives a gentle stretch to the lower back. Lower leg and repeat on other side. With your partner lying on their front, lift the leg.

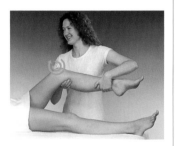

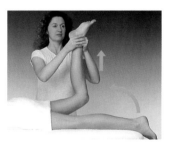

2 Bend the knee, moving the leg upward and, while supporting the back of the knee with one hand and the ankle with the other, rotate the hip joint, making small circles with the knee.

4 Holding the ankle in both hands, lift the foot up toward the ceiling, bending the leg at the knee. Lift and lower the leg gently, giving a gentle stretch to the front of the thigh and the front of the hip.

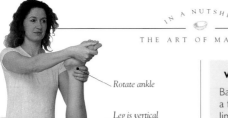

Rotate ankle

Leg is vertical

5 Still holding the ankle at
right angles to the body, let
the knee now rest on the table
and shake the foot. Holding the
ankle with one hand and the
middle of the foot with the other,
rotate the ankle joint, first in one
direction and then back in the
other. Grasp toes with one hand,
flex them forward and then curl
them gently back. Lower heel
gently downward toward buttock
as far as is comfortable, to give a
slightly stronger stretch to the
front of the thigh. Lower leg to
the table.

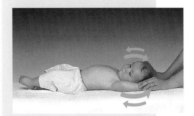

- Holding the baby's hands, lift
both arms and stretch them
outward and in, and then up
above the head and back down
to the side again.

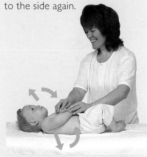

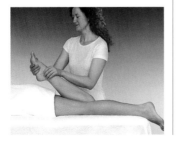

- Cross the arms over chest,
open the arms gently out to the
side, and then cross them in
front of the chest once more.

Contraindications

In general, massage is an extremely safe form of therapy; however, there are some situations where massage should be avoided.

These include:
- AIDS (where there are cuts or lesions).
- Areas of local infection (e.g. shingles, ringworm, athlete's foot).
- Bruising (never work directly over a bruised area).
- Eczema (weeping).
- Fever or high temperatures.
- Full stomach – always allow at least an hour between eating a meal and receiving massage.
- Heart conditions.
- Menstruation (some schools suggest no massage during the first two days). In practice be much, much gentler over the abdomen.
- Nausea.
- Open cuts or sores.
- Pregnancy (some schools suggest no massage during the first three months). In practice just be much, much gentler on the lower back and avoid the abdominal area.
- Recent major operation.
- Recent scar tissue.
- Swelling or inflammation.
- Thrombosis or phlebitis (painful clot in vein).
- Tumors, or undiagnosed swellings.
- Varicose veins – especially when the veins are painful or swollen.

Self-help for common ailments

THE POWER *of massage is largely due to the positive effect it has on the entire body mechanism, improving the body's general resistance to disease, producing a feeling of well-being, and encouraging the body's innate ability to heal itself. There are, however, a variety of specific problems that massage can help relieve.*

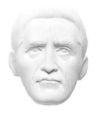

ABOVE **Massage can help soothe many** *disorders associated with the pace of life today.*

Massage can be used either to soothe and relax or to stimulate and revitalize. It is particularly effective for any stress-related disorders such as tension, anxiety, headaches, muscle pains, sleeplessness, depression, and digestive disorders, and its gentle healing properties are equally effective on ailments ranging from babies' colic to the painful arthritis of the elderly.

ABOVE **The feeling of** *well-being engendered by massage may boost the immune system.*

SPECIAL NOTE

A gentle massage can be extremely beneficial to those with cancer, according to recent research which shows that it can help them to relax and feel better. It is, however, inadvisable to massage over the actual site of the cancer.

Any patient, however mild or serious their condition (see page 13 for cautions), can benefit from the healing effects of massage. The mere art of touch itself combined with a caring attitude will be immensely therapeutic. Obviously there are times and situations where an in-depth massage would be inappropriate or just too exhausting: instead a gentle hand massage or a simple face massage using the lightest of strokes can serve to soothe and relax. For anyone who is seriously ill or has recently undergone surgery, always make sure you have the physician's consent first.

OTHER FORMS OF MASSAGE

Aromatherapy (which involves the use of plant essences) and shiatsu (an Eastern pressure technique) are both massage-based therapies, involving diagnosis and definitive treatment. They are therefore specifically structured to treat certain ailments and diseases as well as working on the body as a whole. You may be interested to investigate techniques for both of these therapies. Visit your library for further information.

ABOVE AND RIGHT **Many plant essences are used in aromatherapy.**

RIGHT **Aromatherapy oils are widely available for purchase and use in the home.**

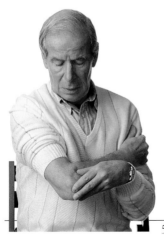

LEFT **The pain of arthritis may be eased by massaging around the affected area.**

Common ailments

MANY CONDITIONS *may be helped by either a full-body massage, or massage of the affected part. This section suggests remedies for many common afflictions, but remember that if you are at all unsure about the advisability of undertaking a massage, consult a physician.*

Alzheimer's disease
A general, all-over body massage can sometimes help relieve the symptoms of this disease.

Anxiety, anxiety attacks
A full-body massage will help soothe, calm and relax the body.

Arthritis and rheumatism
Massage gently above and below the affected area, then, with light, gentle strokes, massage the whole area. Direct the strokes upward and toward the heart.

> **CAUTION**
>
> If you are suffering from a painful condition or if symptoms persist, remember to consult your physician.

Babies' ailments
Colic, restlessness, and insomnia can be helped by regular gentle massage.

Back pain
Massage the whole of the back, neck, legs, feet, and abdomen to reduce pain and relieve tension.

Bereavement
A soothing full-body massage, using flowing rhythmic strokes, helps comfort and relax the sufferer.

Bronchitis
Massage the upper back, chest, and neck to help reduce tension, stimulate the circulation to the area, improve respiration, and clear the chest.

Bruises
Do not work directly over the bruise: instead work above any area of bruising, toward the heart, to speed healing.

Catarrh
Massage the face, neck, and shoulders to release tension and encourage sinus drainage.

Chilblains
Regular massage will stimulate the circulation and help to reduce the symptoms. Massage also works preventively so if you are prone to chilblains, whole-body massage, paying particular attention to the extremities, will be helpful.

Constipation
Massage the lower back and then the abdomen, slowly circling the area in a clockwise direction using light strokes to begin with and then gradually working more firmly.

Coughs (including asthma)
Massage to the back and the neck will release tension and as a result will improve breathing.

Cramp
Massage the affected area to release muscle tension.

Depression
A soothing full-body massage, using flowing rhythmic strokes, will lift the spirits and dispel depression.

Digestive problems
Massage the abdomen gently in a clockwise movement, followed by the lower back. This will help release any tension and encourage the digestive process.

Elderly people's ailments
Common problems such as stiffness in joints, lack of mobility, poor circulation, poor digestion, and sleeplessness can all be helped by regular body massage. Massage the affected area,

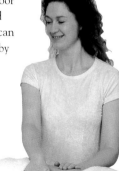

working toward the heart.
Full-body massage will
revitalize, and ease complaints.

Exhaustion, lack of energy
A full-body massage will improve
circulation, relax and revitalize
the body.

Eyestrain
Massage the face, head, and neck
to relax the whole area, paying
particular attention to the area
around the eye socket and the
base of the skull, where eyestrain
may cause a build-up of tension.

Foot pain, bunions
Gently massage the feet to
improve flexibility and release
tension. A little oil will help to
soften hardened skin.

Headaches
Massage the back, neck, face,
and head to relieve pain and
reduce muscle tension.

Heart disease
The soothing effects of massage
can help reduce levels of stress,
calming the entire mechanism.
Consult your physician before
undergoing treatment.

High blood-pressure
General body massage can relax
the body and encourage lowering
of the blood-pressure.

Hyperventilation
General massage can help relax
the body, reducing anxiety and
calming the breathing.

Infant colic
Gently massage the abdomen in
a clockwise direction and the
back to release muscle spasm,
improve the digestion and calm
your baby. Use a little Roman
chamomile essential oil in a light
carrier oil (see page 19) to soothe
and relax.

Insomnia
Massage the whole body or the
back, as late in the
day as possible. Use
gentle, rhythmic
strokes to relax
and soothe.
Finish the
massage by
stroking lightly
down the spine,
one hand
following
the other.

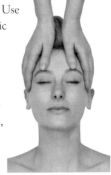

Irritable bowel syndrome
Massage the mid-back and abdomen to relax tension and soothe the whole area. A full-body massage or head and shoulders massage will be useful 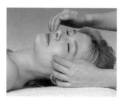 during periods of stress which tend to exacerbate this condition.

Jaw problems (clenched, painful)
Massage the face, head, and neck, encouraging the sufferer to relax the face as much as possible. Pay particular attention to the jaw muscle itself.

Menstrual disorders
Massage the abdomen and lower back to relax the body and release tension.

Migraine
Massage the mid-back, shoulders, neck, head, and face, paying particular attention to the area around the eyes. The extent of the massage that you are able to do will depend upon the severity of the migraine and the sufferer's resulting sensitivity.

Muscular aches
Massage the affected area to reduce pain and relax muscle tension.

Pain
Massaging the whole body, or massaging around the affected area, can help relax the body and relieve pain.

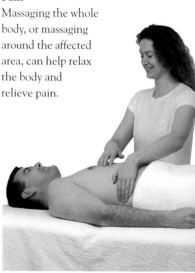

Palpitations
In cases where this condition is stress-related, regular, gentle body massage will relax and soothe the sufferer.

Parkinson's disease

Regular massage can help calm the nervous system, improve circulation, enhance well-being and encourage a positive body image.

Poor circulation

General body massage can help stimulate and improve the blood circulation. Work toward the heart whenever possible.

Postural problems

General body massage can help to release chronic muscle tension and help to undo old habits which have resulted in bad posture.

Pregnancy ailments

For poor circulation, and back pain resulting from poor posture, massage the whole of the back area, paying particular attention to the middle of the back. Insomnia, morning sickness (massage with a little ginger essential oil), and varicose veins will also respond to massage.

RSI (repetitive strain injury)

Regular massage to the back, neck, head, arms, and hands will ease muscular tension and improve the circulation.

Shoulder pain, frozen shoulder

Massage the shoulder area, the upper back, chest, and neck to improve mobility and release tension, helping to relieve the pain.

Skin problems

General body massage can improve poor circulation and lymphatic drainage (drainage of toxins from the body) and improve skin tone, dryness, and elasticity.

Sleep problems

Sleep disorders and restlessness can be helped by regular, soothing massage, which is particularly useful an hour or so before bed. Combine with some relaxing aromatherapy oils, like lavender and chamomile. Adult insomniacs may respond to marjoram essential oil, but this is not suitable for children.

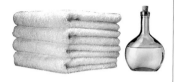

Sprains

Gentle massage can speed up the healing process. An ice pack or cold compress should be applied to the swelling. Then gently massage above and below the injury to encourage waste fluids to drain away.

Strains

Gentle massage of the strained area can help relieve pain and speed up the healing process.

Stress

General massage can help reduce the negative effects of stress to both the body and the mind, soothing, relaxing, and recharging the entire mechanism.

Teething problems

Babies and children may suffer from symptoms when first and second teeth appear, and massage can be very useful to soothe and balance. Massage the abdomen, back, neck, and face to relax the child and reduce muscle tension and pain.

Tennis elbow

Massage over tender spot on elbow, and down the arm. Consult your physician before undergoing treatment.

Tension

Full-body massage can help relax and restore the body.

Varicose veins

Avoid massaging directly over varicose veins: massage gently above them, working toward the heart to encourage drainage. Hold the affected area between the hands in order to soothe and encourage healing.

Further reading

AROMATHERAPY: AN A–Z by *Patricia Davis* (C.W. Daniel, 1988)

THE BOOK OF MASSAGE by *Lucinda Lidell* (Ebury Press, 1958)

AROMATHERAPY by *Judith Jackson* (Dorling Kindersley, 1987)

THE COMPLETE BOOK OF MASSAGE by *Clare Maxwell-Hudson* (Dorling Kindersley, 1988)

THE MASSAGE BOOK by *George Downing* (Penguin, 1974)

THE COMPLETE ILLUSTRATED GUIDE TO MASSAGE by *Stewart Mitchell* (*Element, 1997*)

SHIATSU: JAPANESE MASSAGE FOR HEALTH AND FITNESS by *Elaine Liechti* (Element, 1992)

MASSAGE: A PRACTICAL INTRODUCTION by *Stewart Mitchell* (Element, 1992)

Useful addresses

UK
School of Complementary Health
38 South Street
Exeter EX4 1ED
Tel: 01392 410 954
www.schoolofcomplementaryhealth.co.uk

Northern Institute of Massage
14-16 St. Mary's Place
Bury
Lancs BL9 0DZ
Tel: 0161 797 1800
www.nim56.co.uk

USA
Boulder School of Massage Therapy
6255 Longbow Drive
Boulder
Colorado
CO 80301
Tel: (800) 442 5131

American Massage Therapy
Association
820 Davis Street
Suite 100
Evanston
Illinois 60201 4444
Tel: (708) 864 0123
www.amtamassage.org

International Massage Association
PO Drawer 421
Warrington
Virginia 20188 0421
Tel: (540) 351 0800
www.ima.org

AUSTRALIA
Society of Clinical Masseurs
PO Box 8060
North Camberwell
Victoria 3124
Australia
Tel: (03) 9817 7577